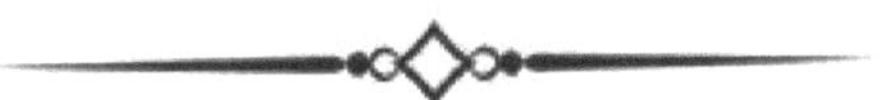

Great works are performed

not by strength

but by perseverance

- Samuel Johnson -

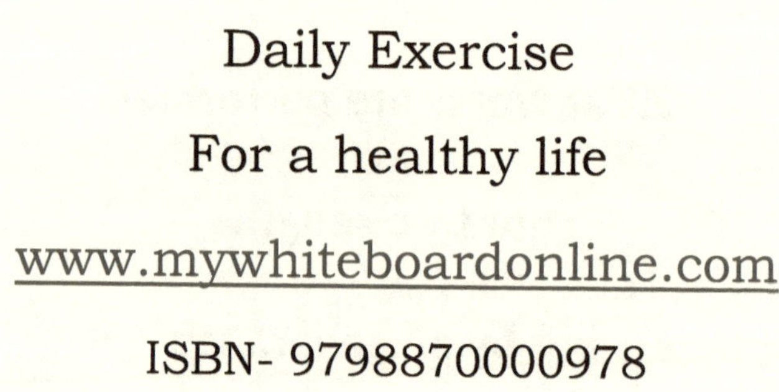

Daily Exercise

For a healthy life

www.mywhiteboardonline.com

ISBN- 9798870000978

Visit www.mywhiteboardonline.com

Set up your activity tracker

to count the number of times an activity

was done in a month and a year

Set up your daystrack

to find the number of days to go

for important events and days

Find the number of days elapsed

since past tasks and events

Set up your mylinks page

to store all your website links in one place!

Shop for products that make a difference

www.mywhiteboardonline.com

<u>How to use the book</u>

The book has three rounds of simple exercises. Each round has seven sessions. Users can do one or more sessions each day. And after they complete three rounds, they can start again from the beginning.

Each Session is a combination of a breathing activity and a simple exercise. You can complete one or more sessions each day and bookmark the page by folding the page. You can then resume the activities the later!

Session one starts with checking the pulse Normal Pulse rate should be 60 to 100 per minute. After that, breath in slowly and breath out slowly for sometime. Then focus on normal breathing for a few minutes! In Session two raise your hands above head and bring it down a few times. Then Hold your breath for some time. Resume normal breathing after that and relax. In Session three, bend front and rise a few times. Then breath in slowly and breath out slowly for sometime. In Session four, open and close your palms a few times. Then hold your breath for a while!

In Session five, stretch your feet for sometime. Then breath in slowly and breath out slowly.

In Session six, rotate your shoulders for sometime. After that, hold your breath for a while. Resume normal breathing after that!

In Session seven, do simple eye exercises by rotating your eyes. Then move eyes from left to right and right to left. Repeat a few times. Breath in slowly and breath out slowly after that!

Combining simple breathing activities with exercises will give extra-ordinary benefits to us. This book can be used by people of all ages. The book can be carried easily and we can devote a few minutes every day to do the exercises given in the book. We can do the activities and bookmark the page and resume the activities later! Surely, this book can help us to do the exercises daily and bring about great changes to our health! And a healthy body and mind can make our life successful and happy!

Check Pulse

Session 1 – Round 1

Breath in slowly

Breath out slowly

After that sit quietly

and focus on

normal breathing

Hands above head

and bring down

Repeat a few times

Hold your breath

for sometime

After that sit quietly

and focus on

normal breathing

Bend front and rise

Repeat a few times

Breath in slowly

Breath out slowly

After that sit quietly

and focus on

normal breathing

Open and close palm

Hold your breath

for sometime

After that sit quietly

and focus on

normal breathing

Feet stretch

Breath in slowly

Breath out slowly

After that sit quietly

and focus on

normal breathing

Rotate shoulders

Hold your breath

for sometime

After that sit quietly

and focus on

normal breathing

Session 7 – Round 1

Eye exercise

Breath in slowly

Breath out slowly

After that sit quietly

and focus on

normal breathing

Session 1 – Round 2

Check Pulse

Breath in slowly

Breath out slowly

After that sit quietly

and focus on

normal breathing

Hands above head

and bring down

Repeat a few times

Session 2 – Round 2

Hold your breath

for sometime

After that sit quietly

and focus on

normal breathing

Bend front and rise

Repeat a few times

Breath in slowly

Breath out slowly

After that sit quietly

and focus on

normal breathing

Open and close palm

Hold your breath

for sometime

After that sit quietly

and focus on

normal breathing

Session 5 – Round 2

Feet stretch

Breath in slowly

Breath out slowly

After that sit quietly

and focus on

normal breathing

Rotate shoulders

Hold your breath

for sometime

After that sit quietly

and focus on

normal breathing

Session 7 – Round 2

Eye exercise

Session 7 – Round 2

Breath in slowly

Breath out slowly

After that sit quietly

and focus on

normal breathing

Check Pulse

Session 1 – Round 3

Breath in slowly

Breath out slowly

After that sit quietly

and focus on

normal breathing

Hands above head

and bring down

Repeat a few times

Hold your breath

for sometime

After that sit quietly

and focus on

normal breathing

Bend front and rise

Repeat a few times

Breath in slowly

Breath out slowly

After that sit quietly

and focus on

normal breathing

Session 4 – Round 3

Open and close palm

Hold your breath

for sometime

After that sit quietly

and focus on

normal breathing

Feet stretch

Breath in slowly

Breath out slowly

After that sit quietly

and focus on

normal breathing

Rotate shoulders

Hold your breath

for sometime

After that sit quietly

and focus on

normal breathing

Eye exercise

Breath in slowly

Breath out slowly

After that sit quietly

and focus on

normal breathing

Four steps of healing

The four steps of healing play a key role in reversing diseases in the human body and in regaining health.

The four basic actions of man are

1) Breathing

2) Eating

3) Thinking

4) Physical actions

Other than congenital diseases, all other disease manifestations occur only when there is a problem with these four basic actions of man.

So, in order to reverse a disease, it is important to adopt a four pronged strategy.

The first step is to correct our breathing.

We have to ensure that we breathe clean and fresh air.

Air is the single most important ingredient of life, and it is important that it has to be clean and pure.

Our health will be greatly enhanced when we breathe clean and fresh air.

We should often go to places like beaches, mountains, rivers and other natural spots to get our dose of fresh air.

It is also a good idea to do yoga and breathing exercises since they regulate the breathing and will bring us very good health benefits.

The second step is to correct our eating.

Next to air, food is the second most important ingredient needed to sustain life. So, it has to be nutritious and healthy. We need to have some basic knowledge of healthy food and follow some simple guidelines regarding food. This is a very key component in maintaining a healthy body.

And the next step is right thinking.

The first two actions are essential for the survival of man and the other two actions contribute to the actual living part of our life.

We live our life by thinking and actions.

And the errors we make in these actions, will have a negative impact on the body, and affect our health. So, it is important to cultivate the habit of positive thinking. We have to make a conscious effort to refrain from negative thoughts. Other than negative thoughts, worrying too much is also a very big stress builder. Worrying a lot will have a big effect on the health of the body.

So, we should practice detaching ourselves from worries and focus on the part that is in our control and act on them to resolve our problems.

And we should also learn to deal with stress, since stress can have a significant impact on our health.

It is essential to learn coping mechanisms to deal with stress.

And if we learn to deal with stress, it leads to immense mental growth. Stress will affect our health only if we handle it wrong.

But if we handle it right, then, it leads to our growth as a human being. In that way, stress plays a very big role in our growth.

The fourth action is physical actions.

We make many errors by resorting to negative habits like smoking, drinking and other activities.

These activities have a very direct effect on the health of the body.

So, it is important to refrain from these negative activities and do more of positive activities like exercise, community work, charity, helping people and other activities. Once we have made a positive lifestyle change by including these activities in our daily routine, our health will be greatly enhanced. And with a healthy body and mind, it is possible to live a meaningful and fruitful life.

Visit www.mywhiteboardonline.com

Set up your activity tracker

to count the number of times an activity

was done in a month and a year

Set up your daystrack

to find the number of days to go

for important events and days

Find the number of days elapsed

since past tasks and events

Set up your mylinks page

to store all your website links in one place!

Shop for products that make a difference

www.mywhiteboardonline.com